The BDSM Code

79 Tips to Turn Your Vanilla Sex Life into a Dungeon Full of Fun

Elizabeth Cramer

The BDSM Code

Publisher: Living Plus Healthy Publishing

ISBN-13: 978-1724733061

ISBN-10: 1724733060

Disclaimer

The Publisher has strived to be as accurate and complete as possible in the creation of this book. While all attempts have been made to verify information provided in this publication, the Publisher assumes no responsibility for errors, omissions, or contrary interpretation of the subject matter herein. Any perceived slights of specific persons, peoples, or organizations are unintentional.

This book is not intended for use as a source of legal, business, accounting or financial advice. All readers are advised to seek services of competent professionals in the legal, business, accounting, and finance fields.

The information in this book is not intended or implied to be a substitute for professional medical advice, diagnosis or treatment. All content contained in this book is for general information purposes only. Always consult your healthcare provider before carrying on any health program.

Table of Contents

Introduction

Sure, you're interested in BDSM and a kinky sex life—who isn't these days? The mainstream media has certainly glamorized the lifestyle recently and the idea of exploring something taboo and erotic definitely gets your heart pounding.

The problem now is, that maybe you're in a committed relationship and can't just go out and find a sub or a Dom to play with. Gee, what a disappointment. All this sexual revolution going on and you're stuck in a vanilla relationship. Maybe you should have experimented with kink back when you were single, right?

Wrong! If anything, being in a committed relationship is the BEST way to improve your sex lives and reach really exciting peaks that you never thought possible. Think about it: you already have established trust with your partner, you already have their respect and their full attention. Now all you have to do is SHOW them how easy and enjoyable experimenting can be. Don't try to sell it, but show them how much fun the two of you could be having.

You can introduce elements of BDSM, role playing and kink into your "vanilla" bedroom, even if you're thinking right about now, "My partner would never go for that!"

Of course that's a natural reaction for a partner that has become accustomed to the routine. He or she may be comfortable where they're at, and not want to do anything too "wild."

But what we're going to show you in this book are tips on how to turn your "vanilla relationship" into something that you both can be excited and passionate about—a "dungeon of fun," so to speak. You really can have the sexy and smoldering relationship you always wanted but never thought possible.

We will cover "troubleshooting" subjects on:

- Explaining BDSM to someone who doesn't understand

- How to remove the stigma of "abusive" sex

- Why sexual kink is nothing to be afraid or ashamed of

- How to help yourself and your partner confront the most taboo of fears and fantasies

- How to repair a sexless marriage

- How to get over fear of your naked body (or your partner's)

- How to be more dominant if you're naturally shy

- And what to do if your kink or your partner's kink is way over the top and freaky

By the end of the book you're going to feel confident about talking to your partner about sex, fantasies and new ideas. We're going to show you how to do it with class, good taste and above all, respect for the good relationship you have going.

Let's get started with Chapter 1, as we explain what BDSM is, to a person who doesn't understand the concept and has negative associations.

Chapter 1: How to Explain BDSM to Someone Who Doesn't Understand

One of the most common reasons couples disagree about kinking up their relationship is because one of the partners doesn't understand "kink" or the BDSM lifestyle at all. One partner may explain BDSM in a sentence, or perhaps in a full conversation, but he or she will only explain it from his/her own perspective.

What you think of something as kinky, hot and interesting, your partner may find it very intimidating. Perhaps you are unaware of how you're making the activity sound. With certain words you use, you may conjure up dark and disturbing imagery in the mind of your partner.

It's not your fault for describing it in a less than spectacular way, nor is it your partner's fault for misunderstanding. It happens...now the solution is to improve communication and better explain what BDSM means to an average couple.

Assuming that anyone who has reservations to kink is probably imagining the worst of the worst. Whatever horror stories they've heard about, they're thinking something along the lines of that. It's up to you to show them that BDSM as an activity doesn't have to be a "lifestyle."

Tip #1: Make it clear to your partner that BDSM means "Bondage & Discipline, Dominance & Submission and Sadism & Masochism" but that most people who enjoy it do NOT do all of the above.

You will find that the people you talk to in the lifestyle usually have one preference and they may not go far beyond that. Some women are very turned on by a dominant lover, but they may not want to be "abused" as with sadism at all. Some men may enjoy being tied up but that doesn't mean they want to be humiliated by their partner.

BDSM activities are simply linked together for convenience purposes, a sort of catch-all label that simply means "non-mainstream" or niche love-making. It's merely a different type of role-playing or love play, with its own unique avenues that you can explore or choose to avoid.

The easiest way to calm your partner's fears is to gauge what exactly they think "kink" involves. Find out what misconceptions they have and then explain the truth of the matter; mainly that BDSM means very different things from one person to another. This is because the term implies sexual exploration and discovery, and that has to be an individual process.

Tip #2: Explain that BDSM or Kink isn't about following a bunch of strange sexual rules. It's about exploring what turns us on as individuals and as a couple. That's all.

If you're trying to initiate your partner into the "lifestyle" then you're going about it the wrong way. It's just like a guy who tries to intimidate and pressure his girlfriend into having a threesome when she obviously doesn't want to do it. No good can come from trying to force, or pressure, someone into the activity.

Even with Dominance and Submission, the goal is not to dominate your partner and establish a bunch of rules to follow.

Tip #3: The goal is to explore what erotic thoughts you have in common with each other and find ways to explore those thoughts.

The minute you start trying to set rules or tell your partner what to do without a process of negotiation and discussion, you're doomed. Consider BDSM a form of sexual therapy, not just a bunch of kinky lists and suggestions. It's not a board game, it's not a club you join. It's a process of discovering who you are, and who your partner is.

Tip #4: BDSM is not always about sex, believe it or not.

If your partner has grim visions of orgies, Satanic rituals and lacerating bodies with bull whips, assure them that's far from what's going to happen. In fact, many people in BDSM activity don't have sex at all. They are after an emotional experience, a catharsis of emotion, oftentimes suppressed from childhood.

Most people—granted, not all—but most people involved in the lifestyle is sane, and probably more sane than the average population, if you believe that sexual repression contributes to neuroses. A kinkster simply explores their sexuality more so than a "vanilla" lover who is satisfied (or not too satisfied) with the standard missionary position.

Tip #5: BDSM is built on the concept of saying No.

In this respect, it is like any other sexual activity, in which one partner suggests something and the other partner has the option to say Yes or No. Most people who are active in the lifestyle read a great deal about the experiences of others (and you're off to a great start!). So what might help is explaining to your partner that there are multiple sources of information and what he or she might have heard may be counteracted by another source of information.

Obviously, if they've only learned about the practice from television or the movies (where Doms are usually portrayed as psychotic) then they have a warped view of the activity, as well as the benefits it has brought many couples over the years.

Tip #6: Remind your partner that BDSM is not really spontaneous fun. It's all about talking and non-romantic agreement and clauses.

The Hollywood or even literate depictions of BDSM paint the activity as exciting and spontaneous, rather than the rather methodical and pre-arranged that it is. Rough sex may work in the movies, but if you take that approach to the real thing, you're going to scare the daylights out of your partner—especially if your spouse has warped perceptions of what BDSM means.

Your partner needs to understand above all else…

Tip #7: BDSM is about your partner, not just you pleasing yourself.

When you make the activity about both you and your partner, then your suggestions will be far less intimidating. He or she will quickly understand that it's a cooperative game, one where you can both set the rules and decide on the direction you want to go. No one has to suffer humiliation or pain, because you operate together as one.

In the next chapter, we're going to introduce you to some concepts that will help you make a better case for BDSM exploration, to a partner who is deadest on opening his/her mind. Let's talk about what dominance really means.

Chapter 2: How to Persuade Your Partner to be Kinky if He or She Dislikes BDSM

To a partner that *decides* he/she doesn't like BDSM or what it stands for, it is going to be an uphill battle to persuade them otherwise. First, it's important that you avoid taking an argumentative stance. The more you try to force or intimidate your partner into doing something he or she doesn't want to do, the more resistance you will face.

BDSM games aside, no one likes a bossy person barking orders or trying to "guilt" them into doing something they don't want to do—it's obscene and degrading.

However, accepting their feelings and respecting their statements doesn't mean you have to give up trying to enjoy a better sex life with your partner.

Tip #8: Stop preaching BDSM. Start thinking about "CONCEPTS" that you and your partner can agree upon.

There's a big difference between saying, "I want us to start doing bondage and discipline together because it turns me on" and "I like the idea of being a dominant lover."

What's the difference? One is intent on manipulating the partner into following his/her lead, whether the partner agrees or not. The other is mostly about feelings that the partner has, and what he can OFFER to his partner in terms of negotiation. He likes to be in control and his partner may be able to work with THAT—but still not call it BDSM.

And that's fine, because BDSM means nothing except sexual exploration. There is no list of rules and it's not a game or a checklist that everyone has to agree upon.

If your partner doesn't like "BDSM" then that means there is a particular avenue or activity that upsets them and conjures up bad feelings. Naturally you avoid that at all cost. But while you avoid calling it BDSM, you can still entertain some of the concepts that are in BDSM, so as long as they are pleasurable and at the speed of your partner.

BDSM in Everyday Life

Here's an example. Let's say a wife has a husband who doesn't like BDSM because he associates it with abuse, perverted sex and spankings. Coming from an abusive home, he does not like the connotations and has closed his mind to BDSM play.

Now the wife, who has all kinds of taboo fantasies, has three options. She can argue with him and try to force him to accept that BDSM is what she wants and he must accommodate her. Two, she can accept his refusal to experiment and be satisfied with a boring sex life. Or three, she can negotiate some compromise between one and two.

She's not going to force him to do anything, but she doesn't have to give up trying to open his mind to new concepts. Instead of calling it BDSM play, a trigger word for her husband, she'll simply tell him what he wants to hear.

"I like it when you take control. I like when you're powerful and dominant."

That really doesn't have anything to do with BDSM rules or kinky sexual experimentation—it's just a personal turn on, and it's something that her husband can appreciate.

Understand that though BDSM has a bad reputation in some conservative circles, much of modern culture embraces these concepts, by any other name. Religious books like the Bible, Torah and Quran all provide illustrations of men being dominant and women being submissive. This is the cornerstone of an active sex life and happy family.

This isn't really a scientific attitude—it's men and women taking a specific role and many people are fine doing it. Some women like being dominated by a confident man. The only real difference is that in BDSM lifestyle, there is equality and women can choose to dominate men, or be dominated in a more blatantly sexual manner.

Whereas some forms of domination might include "loving one's wife and providing discipline," another might be treating a wife like a sexual object, and being a little rough with her. If the wife enjoys one, or the other, or both, that is something the couple can explore.

No matter the case, the common denominator is that all of these activities involve playing roles that make the male and female partner happy. So if one partner does not like BDSM because of one "scenario," then by all means change the scenario.

And if you realize what the problem really is, you can certainly help your partner to open their mind to new activities in general, even if you're not being a traditional "Dom." It's all about finding and respecting each other's boundaries.

Tip #9: If your partner doesn't like certain concepts or plays, then by all means avoid them. But don't let that stop your resolve to FIND SOMETHING your partner likes.

If he or she doesn't like flogging or name calling then that certainly doesn't mean you might as well give up and go full vanilla. It just means you have to work a little harder to find something naughty and exciting that you both enjoy—and again, stop calling it BDSM, because obviously your partner doesn't like that!

Tip #10: Pay closer attention to your partner and learn to read them.

Chances are, if your partner has decided that all BDSM is evil or abusive then you lost their trust at some point in the conversation. Maybe they started out as indifferent and open to the idea, and then somewhere down the line of your conversation, they dropped out and became opposed.

Was it something you said? That's why it's important to gauge their interest and take verbal and non-verbal cues as to their feelings on certain subjects. If they seem put off by graphic language or demeaning words, then are you taking note of their reaction?

A partner doesn't always say "NO" (even though they should) but if they are making faces or gestures that indicate defensiveness, then mark this down as a hard or soft limit that you must tread on carefully.

Remember that non-verbal gestures can be telling, especially about activities they are undecided upon. These signals might include:

- Nervous fidgeting

- Loss of eye contact or squinting

- Looking around the room as if asking, "is anyone else hearing this crazy talk?"

- Biting lips or touching the fact in discomfort

- Folding arms

- Leaning away from you

These gestures can tell you if your partner is starting to lose enthusiasm for what you're suggesting and in that case it's time to back-track and start finding points of agreement once again.

In the next chapter, we're going to discuss why it's important that you and your partner be on the same page, especially for some rather cathartic sexual scenes that may uncover strong hidden emotion that you didn't know you had. Let's proceed with caution.

Chapter 3: How to Help Your Partner Get over Taboo Fears

Our instincts are to clam up when our partners don't cooperate, but this can be troubling to a relationship. The problem is, when one partner gets in tune with their wants and needs they open up a sort of Pandora's Box of explosive sexual feelings they want to explore. It can become an obsession and this is the time to HELP a partner and guide them through this experience.

To simply ignore a partner who is intent on experiencing sexual release is dangerous. Whether you debate the ethics of pressuring a partner to indulge your kinks or not is not the point; the point is if you don't get release from your partner, you will be tempted to get it from someone else. Hopefully you can resist the impulse, but the sex or emotional release you want is a "force of nature," not just a silly passing thought. And the same is true of your partner's needs and your decision on whether to help them or ignore them.

Sexual fantasies can be intensely alluring and the best way to deal with it is for partners to talk to each other and do something about it. That doesn't mean succumbing to pressure, nor does it mean doing something strange and scary. It's about negotiating a solution and creating a fantasy or a scene both partners can enjoy.

Tip #11: Start the conversation by openly confessing what you are attracted to and then listening to what your partner finds attractive.

This is the naked communication process and it has nothing to do with turning your partner on or indulging your own feelings. It is just about honesty and intimacy. This will be a rush of different sorts; not adrenaline but eroticism and relief. Usually your partner will accept your feelings, because believe it or not, most fantasies that people have are not that terrible. (Read on in later chapters just in case yours are!)

Most of these taboo fantasies involve situations so familiar, they are basically mainstream. Whether it's a non-consent fantasy, dirty-talking, rough sex, cheating, older lovers, teacher-student, blackmail, or sex with a stranger, they are all recurring thoughts that all people have.

So when you confess them to your partner, it's not really a big deal in theory — it's just the shock of hearing each other admit, "Wow, I really do think about having sex with people other than you."

And even that is not a big deal, and it certainly doesn't mean the end of your relationship, NOR that you're going to be having threesomes and taking part in orgies. It's just an honest confession. You can both use these abstract thoughts, and build on them, to create a more interesting sex life.

Tip #12: The confession stage is not about being vulgar or overtly sexual. Don't be theatrical, don't be seductive, just be honest.

Of course your partner is not going to like everything you mention and no, not every fantasy will be fulfilled. In fact, now is not the time to elaborate on the fantasy. That's later; for now, just be honest in admitting.

Tip #13: Focus on WHAT your fantasy is and WHY you find it arousing.

For example, the husband starts with confession. He says he admits he's always had hot teacher fantasies. He admits crushes he had, and theorizes that the power that teachers have over students may be what attracts him to the fantasy. She confesses that she has cheating fantasies. She finds the idea of sneaking around and the risk of getting caught very sexy.

There you go, both fantasies are shared and neither partner has any reason to fear, since these are fairly normal fantasies.

It is important that you confess your fantasies with a certain level of class and maybe even restraint, so that you don't speed through the process and make your partner uncomfortable. Don't describe your hot threesome fantasy in a spa just because your partner asked. Take it slow. Start with the idea itself and see how your partner reacts.

Tip #14: Avoid casting blame when speaking your taboo confessions.

This is not about fulfilling your needs or anyone's "failure." Reassure your partner that all of this is based on love.

A sensitive vanilla partner may read into your fantasies so it's important to be communicative and to speak in a loving voice. Reassure them that this doesn't mean you're going to cheat, stop loving them, or force them to do anything. Admit that you were afraid to confess and afraid that he/she wouldn't love you anymore.

This is especially important if your partner seems angry at your confession. Tell them it was hard to be open about your secret shame but that you wanted to be completely honest with him or her. Tell them how you trust your partner enough to do this, whereas previous lovers did not have the same privilege or trust. Usually, your partner will be impressed at your honesty. And besides, you didn't even cheat or hide secrets.

This is the first step in building a stronger relationship. If you explain it in loving terms to your partner, they will accept it.

Tip #15: Answer all questions and ask questions about where the fetish or kink comes from.

Now that you've admitted some familiar and maybe even shocking things, talk about where the feelings of taboo come from, ask questions and answer questions.

Be prepared to hear things like, "what have you done to find out about your fetishes?", as your partner may be suspicious as to what you've already done, and whether you've cheated or not. Don't get upset or taking any of the confession process too personally.

The first step is to let your partner love you, and vice versa, simply knowing of the taboo attraction and accepting it. Accepting it doesn't always mean endorsing it, or allowing you to act completely without restraint.

Tip #16: Before you start creating fantasies, watch movies or read erotica on the taboo topics as a couple.

This will give you the opportunity to live vicariously through others rather than commit to anything yourself. Give your partner an opportunity to see why this taboo is so exciting; let them see someone else speak of its eroticism.

This vicarious experience teaches your partner to view BDSM activity as recreational and perhaps even non-sexual—it lets them know you're still the same person they love and this is just a form of fun and pleasure, like any other sensual activity. It's not a "lifestyle" or a change in your personality.

The next phase will be creating fantasies for each other, either through talking or writing (if you prefer). This is where you can both experiment with the taboos and indulge each other.

Tip #17: Create hard and soft limits.

Creating hard and soft limits is important and not just for your own knowledge, but so that your partner can feel safe. Without boundaries your partner may feel intimidated to carry on.

Hard limits create boundaries that he/she knows you will never cross; this gives your partner the confidence to explore within a comfortable range.

As you develop your new and improved relationship, you may change your soft or hard limits. As trust increases, your partner may turn some soft limits into more explorable territory. But this is progress you must earn.

Try though you might to be creative and flexible in role playing, sometimes a person just makes up their mind that they do not want to try anything new and that they'd rather have no sex life at all than compromise their standards. If that's the case, y ou are stuck between a rock and a hard place for sure. This is the focus of the next chapter, because we believe you should never give up hope!

Chapter 4: What to Do If Your Partner Doesn't Seem to Want Sex at All

It is possible that your partner may reject all your creative ideas entirely and leave you confused and frustrated. First of all, don't give up! Don't conclude that just because your partner isn't feeling it right now, his or her attitude might not change in the future.

First, understand that it's not normal for a partner to be totally uninterested in exploring their sexuality. It's not a matter of, "What can I do about my partner who is failing in his/her responsibility?" It's a matter of, "What can I do to help my partner?"

What obstacle is in the way of a good and healthy relationship? By approaching the problem with a better attitude, a more constructive attitude, you may be able to help your partner overcome their aversion to a more interesting sex life.

Tip #18: Don't blame him or her for the lack of sex or satisfaction. Instead, make them feel safe.

Blaming the partner is just going to put your partner on the defensive. What sometimes happens is that one partner starts building a "case" against the sexually lagging partner and makes their "flaws" the point of the conversation. This is very damaging, since it corrupts what should be a trustful relationship and makes it cynical. Soon, all you can think of is your partner's flaws. This will distort your view of them and only result in more intense arguments.

Instead, try approaching your partner in a spirit of vulnerability. Be honest, compassionate and open-minded. The key is to NOT to put them on the defensive but to make them feel safe and give them the opportunity to improve sexual matters between you two.

Tip #19: Ask yourself if you could be unknowingly contributing to the sexual hangup.

A lot of people may be surprised to find that their behavior—usually not done on purpose—may be putting the other partner on the defensive. Examine your partner's behavior. Is there a correlation between something you do or say, and the negative behavior from your partner?

An objective analysis of your own behavior may reveal that you have the tendency to nag, be passive aggressive, condescending, easily distracted, complaining and so on. Could you improve in listening?

The best way to change a relationship dynamic that seems rocky (and thus almost always has sexual problems or incompatibility) is to identify the negative patterns. Sometimes the negative patterns come from you and in ways you might not expect.

For instance, sometimes a partner will respond to your actions, because you unknowingly cause them to react. A common scenario: a husband tends to talk down to his wife when the subject of sexual fetishes comes up. The wife senses his tone and so she pulls back and clams up. He senses this and becomes more needy and complaining. This makes her even more critical and unwilling to share.

The next thing you know, the wife has banned all creative sexual practices because communication has already broken down. There's no way to open trust levels for new intimate experiences until the damage is repaired.

Tip #20: Don't discuss sexual incompatibility when you're upset.

This should go without saying, but many couples unfortunately still "negotiate" while they're yelling at each other. Waiting until you both simmer down will work to your advantage and let you actually listen to what your partner is afraid of, and why he or she might not want to go too far out in sexual adventure.

Be compassionate, even if you are disappointed with a partner's choice not to try something you find arousing. Your partner is probably feeling vulnerable and afraid at something to do with the BDSM practice being discussed. He or she needs to say NO, to maintain control over their life. They want to feel personal power and hold onto their emotional resilience. It probably has nothing to do with you at all. It's about THEM.

Let them maintain control and have the right of refusal because if they are "forced" or pressured into cooperating they lose all sense of who they are. They lose trust in you.

What you can do, if you continue to feel frustration, is talk to your partner about the way you feel. Be honest and admit that you are feeling frustrated or whatever other emotions you struggle with, because of the lack of sexual compatibility you feel.

It's not a fun conversation, but if you go about it respectfully and with a view towards EXPLAINING YOURSELF, rather than placing blame, your partner will probably give it some serious thought.

Now it's possible your partner will never change their opinion on certain types of activities that feel wrong or hurtful. This is a bit of a crossroads, since you must decide whether to accept his/her limitations. Some BDSM "lifestylers" have left their vanilla spouses because the sex, or role playing, was just that important to them. They were not getting what they wanted and so they ended the relationship.

This is not going to be most people. And rest assured, your partner may be afraid of this scenario happening; hence it's important to reassure them right about now. You just want to expand the menu of sexual options, but you have no intention of leaving or cheating.

While it is true at some point you do have to decide to be content with a relationship without kink (or the kind of kink you long for) it doesn't necessarily mean the end of your sex life.

What is Desire Discrepancy?

One thing that might help you get through this difficult phase of incompatibility is to learn what desire discrepancy is. Outside of BDSM, it is frequently discussed among sex therapists and their patients. One partner is always sexually aggressive and hungry while the other is content with little to no sex, maybe only once a month or so.

There are two options, and realistically, neither of them involve "just dealing with it" because obviously that's going to leave the very horny partner frustrated.

Tip #21: The couple can negotiate and decide on what they have permission to do—with or without each other.

Honesty is important here. The couple who has mismatched libido must negotiate a compromise; usually with one partner seeking out erotic fulfillment from porn, erotica, sex toys or other one-person options.

Some couples decide that it's okay if one partner masturbates in private, using whatever stimuli he/she can get, since the other partner is busy or uninterested in sex at that time.

While this is not as effective as coming up with a more creative compromise, it may be the last resort to a couple that do not want to ignore the problem, but are too afraid to consider more extreme options.

Speaking of extreme options, that would involve option 2: outsourcing a partner's sexual needs to another person, outside of the committed relationship. The couple establishes rules as to the swinging or open marriage arrangement and then welcomes somebody into their bedroom who abides by the rules.

This may involve letting one spouse have sex with another person, or inflicting punishment on them. It's up to the couple to determine if the other partner will watch, join or choose to be absent.

These open relationships are not to be toyed with and frankly are for "advanced" BDSM or swinging members. Couples who have done this kind of thing before and who have unusually high degrees of trust, love and compassion can do it fairly easy—but there are many couples that cannot handle the jealousy.

Let's consider two compromises made in negotiation.

Case 1: One partner decides that she needs BDSM punishment in her life. She wants to be spanked and manhandled. She loves the adrenaline rush she gets from it. Her husband doesn't like it.

Case 2: One partner is aching to have sex with another woman. She doesn't want to share her partner but understands his desire.

For Case 1, the couple decides that the woman can find a boyfriend that will spank her on a regular basis. However, the man sets ground rules: no intercourse. He reveals that he might be jealous if another man were to penetrate her. He only allows spanking and maybe oral sex. The woman agrees and the couple pursues a boyfriend together. There is no cheating involves, since everyone enters into the arrangement honestly.

Case 2: The wife says she cannot bear to share her lover. However, she understands that he craves sex more often than her. So she offers a compromise that he can fantasize, watch porn or read erotica, or role play chat online. Since the husband knows he doesn't want to actually cheat or end the marriage, he agrees to the compromise. The husband finds an outlet for his libido, while the wife doesn't have to feel guilty for holding the husband back from his passions. It may not be the perfect fix, but it's a start and maybe the wife can make an effort to watch porn or read erotica, to up her libido so she can better match her husband.

Thus far, we've talked mostly about your partner's sexual hang-ups but it's now time to direct the attention back on YOU. You never know how your own attitudes and signals may be affecting the relationship. Let's proceed onto Chapter 5.

Chapter 5: How to Get Over Your Taboo Fears

Sometimes you or your partner may be afraid of the very thing you want the most. This happens frequently inside and outside of the kinkster lifestyle, because people crave something subconsciously but can't admit it to themselves.

Usually this results from suppression, guilt, or perhaps even ambivalence as to whether they WANT it or not. Some people just want to fantasize about it. Others crave sexual gratification but are so afraid of actually achieving it that they ruin their chances by doing something contrary to their goal.

This can even happen with couples dabbling into BDSM. For example, a couple wants to swing with other people, but ends up fighting and squabbling over petty jealousies whenever the opportunity comes up.

This is why an important step is, quite simply…

Tip #22: Decide that you actually want to enjoy this kink in reality.

This sounds deceptively simple but a lot of people who fantasize about doing something kinky, cannot bring themselves to do it—even if opportunity comes their way. This means they desire it internally but have reservations about doing it in reality BECAUSE of possible repercussions, whether emotional or physical.

They may fear what successfully fulfilling their fantasy will do to them or their partner. Will it awaken an addiction in them? Will the guilt eat them up inside?

They must decide if they are content with the fantasy or the eroticism is too intense and is begging for a real life experience.

If you and your mate decide that you really want to do something taboo and exciting, then it's important to…

Tip #23: Prepare your life for it, as if you have already accomplished your fantasy.

Visualizing your fantasy "in reality" is the next step. You must prepare your body and mind for the experience you both fear and desire. Imagine the physical reality of what will occur and how other people may react. Talk these over with your partner and get some vivid details down so you can better visualize it happening.

When it finally does happen, you will have imagined it in so much detail that you will be more confident and know what to say or do.

If it helps, you can write yourself dialog to memorize or watch porn or read erotica of similar fantasies and see how those "characters" react in an erotic situation. If you feel socially awkward about it, just imitate the people who are successful.

If you want a more realistic visual, rather than accepting the over-dramatized encounters of erotic entertainment, you might talk to someone who has already done the activity in question, such as an orgy, or a master-slave relationship. Ask them about some of the little details that they should know.

Tip #24: Determine what specifically you are afraid of and then make a plan of action.

Sometimes you're not actually afraid of the fantasy itself, but of possible consequences stemming from it. For example, you love the idea of being a sexual voyeur but the thought of being caught and humiliated is terrifying.

Now that you know what you're afraid of specifically, you and your partner can create a plan of action, taking preventive steps so that you won't encounter that nightmarish scenario.

For instance, if the fear is getting caught then you will plan on camping somewhere, where there aren't many people out and it's unlikely you will get caught. Or perhaps, finding another couple who enjoy being watched.

If you desire to share your bed with a third person, but have a fear of meeting a psychopath or a drug addict, then create a filtering system so you can eliminate the wrong type of lover before ever getting involved with them.

Tip #25: Practice with your partner or by yourself.

Practice could involve physical sexuality or even emotional cues. If you're a man and want to be better in rough sex, but fear losing your erection too soon, then practice masturbating and "edging" without full ejaculation. Improve your stamina with practice.

Practice with your partner talking, and role playing, ever closer to the fantasy. If you fantasize about having sex with a stranger and want to make that a reality in your life, then practice with your willing partner; pretend as if you're meeting each other for the first time. Or, practice making small talk with strangers to remind yourself of how to relate to others on a friendship level—not just a sexual level.

As you've figured out by now, the "taboo" is entirely in your mind. It's up to you to decide whether you want more, or are too squeamish to seek it out as a reality. Your partner can help you with this too.

Tip #26: Ask your partner to "push" you a little bit and help you face your fears.

If your partner is also working towards a common goal of fulfilling your fantasy, this is far more motivating.

If you and your partner agree on a hot fantasy and want to make it as real as possible, then that's double the motivation to actually do it. Your partner can play your "doctor" and help devise ways to take small steps towards the attraction you feel. You can approach it gradually, one tiny step at a time, to calm yourself and not become afraid. In a supportive arrangement with your partner, you should have no fear about accomplishing it.

One reason why partners sometimes clam up for kinkier activities is because of shyness and poor body image in particular. This is both a physical and emotional issue and it's important to approach it as such, as we'll read in the next chapter.

Chapter 6: How to Help Your Partner Overcome a Poor Body Image

One of the most unfortunately common problems in a lack of sexual excitement is that one or both of the partners feels self-conscious about their body. Since BDSM is often associated with high confidence and performance, shy people may literally be afraid of being naked.

They may be comfortable being naked on their own or even in traditional sexual positions—especially with the lights off. But when it comes to real BDSM experience and showing confidence in sexual positions, they just can't do it.

This is known as poor body image. Of course, porn and Hollywood sexy movies don't help matters since everyone is gorgeous and to unrealistic proportions. An even great-

er problem though is that one (or both) partners just don't feel comfortable in their own
skin.

It's not just love handles or fat either. Some
people are very self-conscious about their
body parts individually; their legs, thighs,
breasts, or even their moles and acne. While
it's easy to tell a person, "Just stop caring what
other people think!", a better solution is to…

**Tip #27: Show your partner that you think
he/she is the sexiest thing on earth!**

Now is the time to be reassuring. Don't be
suspiciously quiet. Don't avoid eye contact
even if you're shy. You have to be the strong
one, since you want more sexual connection
and more unique experiences.

Remember that it's the flaws of a person
that really make us stand out from all the others. Tell your partner he/she looks beautiful,
sexy and respond emotionally and deeply to
their body. Encourage them, even if you think
that it's over the top. That's what your partner
needs to hear right now.

Tip #28: The both of you should spend time playing with yourself.

One of the most powerful experiences a shy person can have is looking at himself or herself in the mirror. Privately, so that they can make peace with what they look like. Pleasuring one's self in front of a mirror can also help the person to see himself (or herself) as a sexual being.

If you or your partner has a history of avoiding eye contact, this is the next step. Encourage each other and take it slow at first. For example, stripping one piece of clothing at a time in the other person's presence. Even if you have to break the small steps down smaller (such as being naked with a towel), it's important to start the process and work your way toward the goal of being naked.

Tip #29: Massage also helps. Rather than just telling your partner you admire their body, touch it—caress, rub and titillate each part.

Avoid the genitals for a while and just focus on giving pleasure to your partner through sensual massage, or if they prefer, an actual massage. This is a way of communicating love for each other's bodies in a non-verbal way. It also helps you make peace with your body (since you're naked too) and the way your hands touch your partner's body. Do this routine regularly until being naked in each other's presence is second-nature.

Tip #30: Learn to laugh.

Having fun is more important than doing everything right.

Part of making peace with your naked bodies involves putting away fears of being a perfect sexual being—even in matters of embarrassing noises. It's true...couples frequently burp, pass gas, queef, cough, sneeze and all sorts of other natural bodily functions. You don't hear about them in movies because, of course, movies are simulated reality—not reality.

And in real life, no one cares about that sort of thing. The idea of being humiliated because of something "breaking the mood" is silly. The only point where you "break the mood" is if you get UPSET about a minor quibble.

If you can laugh it off and continue on IN THE MOOD, then there's no reason to feel humiliated. The funny thing came and went and now it's back to the eroticism you crave.

By getting all upset about it and picking a fight with your partner (or doing the opposite and clamming up in embarrassment) you only defeat yourself. Your partner shouldn't care, neither should you.

If she is naturally shy, then it's up to you to teach her to laugh it off. It's okay to laugh and it's okay to blush. But help her understand that fixating on the flaws—which are just real life happening—are not the opposite of sexy. They're real. They're good. Enjoy the reality of a good sex life and whatever you do don't scowl the whole time. Learn to laugh and make it fun for your partner.

How to Help Your Partner Overcome Shyness

Some types of shyness are not really physical but entirely mental and emotional. For instance, what about the partner that is afraid of failing? While sex is pretty easy, vanilla sex that is, the idea of "failing" at being a Dominatrix or a good sub could be intimidating.

Tip #31: The solution lies in teaching your partner how to act, how to react and how to remain calm and in control.

If you want to teach your partner to be a good Dom or sub, then by all means train them. Granted, it's a bit harder to teach a naturally shy person to be a Dom, but you can still give them pointers about how to take control and let their inhibitions go.

For one thing, focus on fulfilling your partner's needs. When you meet new lovers in BDSM, your focus is always in pleasing your new partner. If you are in a relationship, take the same attitude.

Make sure you START with activities she likes. If she's a shy sub, start by lightly spanking or lightly pleasuring her. Get her (or him) used to the mood, and to the scene, but use very light foreplay.

This will gradually help her to release her fear, while also letting the both of you know what she responds to.

Tip #32: Focus on creating a no-pressure environment.

This is equally as important as letting your partner feel safe and sexy. If your partner feels pressured to orgasm, or to make you orgasm, or be a perfect Dom/sub, it's going to be overwhelming.

This means that it may even stress your partner out that he/she can't orgasm on command. For example, some women become so anxious they mentally block themselves from orgasming. Just the same, men can become so nervous about performance anxiety that they become impotent.

All of this is silly—sex and BDSM fun should be enjoyed regardless of stamina, orgasm, goals and scores. Sex should happen because it's pleasurable and it doesn't matter if a person comes or chooses not to.

Emphasize to your partner it doesn't matter if they orgasm or not because all that's important is that you have fun—regardless of a goal…in fact, that's why we recommend this.

Tip #33: Eliminate the need for orgasm for at least two or three sessions.

Don't orgasm—either one of you. Explore each other's bodies without the need to "finish."

This will not only help your partner to feel safer and more secure, but will also train the both of you to be more sensual and more attune to each other's bodies beyond the orgasm phase. Learn to listen to your partner's body and feel what they feel with each shared touch.

The fear of disappointing YOU is what your partner is most afraid of, in many cases. Keep that in mind and focus on being a better lover rather than a strict Dom, at least for the time being.

Affirmations also work very well with self-conscious lovers who need constant reminders that they are doing well. Flatter their ego a bit and let them feel uninhibited—as if nothing they can possibly do will kill the mood. You welcome his/her free and natural self.

Tip #34: Tell them how they should feel.

If your partner is especially shy or with-drawn, more affirmations may be needed, in-cluding confidence building mantras such as "You're not going to feel embarrassed. There's nothing to worry about," or something simi-larly affirming. In this case you are not just encouraging them but using hypnotic lan-guage to influence their feelings.

That brings us to a touchy subject: what if you're the one supposed to be confident and reassuring but you're still shaking in your (leather) boots? That's what we'll discuss in the next chapter.

Chapter 7: How to Be a Dom if You Are Shy, Introverted or Have Low Self-Esteem

Great question and just because you aren't a naturally dominant or extroverted person doesn't mean you can't learn—especially if your partner is going to rely on your show of confidence.

Being a dominant lover simply means being more alpha in personality. In wolf-pack theory, alphas are leaders. They are aggressive, powerful and can communicate effectively. Omegas and betas are their subordinates and they follow the leader.

Perhaps your instincts are to "follow" and try to please your partner, maybe even altering your natural voice and temperament when you do. It's time to change that, at least for this BDSM experiment.

Tip #35: Focus not on being alpha but on NOT being omega.

One of the best ways to fight your instincts to be shy and withdrawn are to watch for your TYPICAL behavior and do the opposite of it. If your natural tendency is to talk softly, then give your voice more power and pitch. If you talk fast when you're nervous then make it a point to slow down and carefully choose your words.

If you have trouble maintaining eye contact then practice with people you meet in everyday life. Look at them and keep eye contact as you speak, for the entire conversation. Notice how it changes the conversation in subtle ways.

Tip #36: The secret to confidence is that you don't "need" what it is you fear losing.

While this makes more sense when you're single and dating, it can still apply to couples in relationships. What you fear losing the most motivates your behavior in ways you don't even realize. Once you realize that you don't need "it" to be happy and survive, your confidence comes back to you.

This is plain to see in courtship, where one person stops being needy and "nice" and focuses instead on being interesting.

In coupling, this means that if one partner is feeling sexually frustrated (sex being the "need") it's time to stop complaining, stop nagging, stop being negative, and instead assume a more confident persona—one who communicates what he/she wants and does so in a positive manner.

Tip #37: A Dom is working FOR the sub. Think about that: that is your motivation.

Contrary to what it might seem, the Dom does not exist because he's there. The Dom exists **because of the sub**, because the sub is the one who wants to be pleased. So in figuring out how to be more confident, try to determine what your partner actually wants.

If your partner is the "sub" meaning he/she gets pleasure from you, determine what turns them on. You can base this on what they've already told you. For example, strong and silent drifters are a turn on for her. This is your "motivation" in being confident; mimicking that type of persona, for her fantasy to come true.

Since you as a Dom exist because of her desires, this is what you become as a more confident lover.

Tip #38: Don't try to take on too much.

The Dom has a lot of responsibility so if you are playing that role, take it slow, especially during negotiation. As exciting as dramatic foreplay sounds, you may actually be giving yourself too much to do, as well as your partner. Take it slow and become more confident in little things before becoming the Dungeon Master of your fantasies.

Most people curious about bondage don't actually start with rope or chains. They start with a blindfold and explore that, working their way up to something kinkier. Keeping things non-threatening and even a little slow is not just good for your partner's sensitivity, but also helps you become a more dominant teacher.

Switch Hitting Tips: How to Play Opposite Your Instincts

When it comes to being a switch, flexible is everything—and we're not just talking body flexible! Whereas some people only prefer to be top or bottom, Dom or sub, the "switch" is a very talented individual who can play both roles. First, understand that many switches do have a preference, and may "substitute" as their opposite role—if for no other reason, than because they do it so well.

So you can definitely have a preference but still be able to assume sub and Dom roles. It can actually be helpful for a person to play both Top and Bottom, as it well help them learn about what their partner desires.

What can occur is that "new" switches can play their role poorly because of confusing messages—which results from not knowing if one is a sub or Dom. This is another reason why it's better to start slow, especially if you and your partner are taking turns in dominant or submissive roles.

Tip #39: Dress for the part.

What frequently happens in BDSM life-style, is that switches dress as a Dom or a sub, depending on who they are seeing. This helps emphasize who they are at that moment and also gives their partner a strong message about how to treat them. The same can be said for couples dabbling into role play.

If you are trying to be more confident, dress like a confident person. A man might want to put on a suit as opposed to casual clothes. A woman may want to dress sexy if she is a sub, or even as a Dominatrix, if she is playing dominant. Wear the clothes from your "real life" that make you feel confident when experimenting.

One nice thing about learning how to "switch" between top and bottom roles is that you can take turns leading and make a game of it; as in getting "revenge" on your partner for the last time they punished you.

Some couples even make a betting game out of it, betting "slave time" as a punishment and creating a list of sexy tasks the partner has to do. If you know that you are mostly going to be dominant with your partner, then it helps to experience the punishment or pleasure you will be giving him or her. It lets you know intimately how each activity feels, giving you better perspective on how to lead.

It's all about honesty and the experience. If you can become a better dominant lover through submissive experience, it will work to play both roles. If you are naturally submissive but want to give your partner pointers on how to be more aggressive then assume the Dom role for educational purposes.

That brings us to our next subject, a rather difficult issue to broach…what if your partner just sucks at being a Dom or a sub?

Chapter 8: What if Your Partner isn't a Very Good Dom or Sub?

This is a rather awkward subject to discuss but frankly, if your partner is a bad Dom or sub it's not the kind of thing you can ignore. The first step is to figure out what's wrong and why they aren't performing the role very well.

Tip #40: First, determine whether it's because they are misguided but sincere or if they really don't care about improving their performance.

If the latter is true then it's back to square one—where has communication broken down? Why are they resisting? Are they afraid of taboos or just resentful at you and thus not willing to try? What can you do to repair the damage of trust? What can you do to help them overcome their fears?

Here's a common scenario in the BDSM lifestyle for newcomers. The man doesn't like the feeling of being a Dom so he wants to be the sub. The woman plays the role of Domme, but he doesn't like the way she does it. When it's her turn to be sub, he just loses all interest in the power play altogether. Do you see what happened here? It was response to a bad relationship dynamic, not really a matter of ignorance.

Tip #41: Figure out what your partner wants and how you can give it to them.

Most partners will want something in exchange for trying to become a better Dom or sub for you. Depending on the stability of your relationship, it may be something minor (like "I don't like aggressive Domination...I like a loving daddy Dom type instead) or it could be much bigger, perhaps about the relationship itself.

Could you improve in some area to make your partner happy and thus be motivated to be a better performer for you? In exchange for your partner being a better Dom, would you be willing to give up something that bothers him or her? Like flirting with other people or chatting to other singles online?

This is just an illustration but it serves the point that trusting each other is about compromise and negotiation. It's not just the sex that's contractual—it's the trust between you that must be drawn up and agreed upon before progress can be made.

You may be surprised at how harder your partner tries, when they see evidence of you working to improve yourself. It's not a one way street, in other words. Both partners have to work at improving the relationship.

Tip #42: If your partner seems confused about how to be a good Dom or sub, then help educate them, without lecturing.

Lecturing your spouse about what they are doing wrong is a bad move and will only worsen communication. Instead, try to suggest ways to improve what is already working. Give them credit for what you do like and then offer pointers on what you want to see more of, and what does NOT work as well.

It always helps to explain "how you feel," how things affect you personally, rather than generalizing the issue.

Saying "No woman likes to be called a slut during sex, treat me with respect!" is a generalization and it only puts your partner on the defensive. Instead, a partner might say, "I don't like name calling because it reminds me of when I was bullied as a teen."

That's something your partner can understand very easily.

Tip #43: Rely on sexualized fiction to illustrate the way a Dom acts.

Your partner may not "know" how Doms behave in movies and books. If he/she is all out of ideas, viewing movies or reading books together can jumpstart his imagination. There are really only four options in "improving" a Dom/sub's performance and this is the first one. This is the least drastic option, as it allows you to address the issue as a couple and take it at a slower pace.

Tip #44: Take on a role reversal and play switch.

Show your partner how your ideal Dom or sub acts to give them concrete examples of dialog and mannerisms. Contrary to popular belief, you don't always have to be a Dom or a sub. And a "switch" doesn't always play 50/50. Sometimes a switch actually prefers to be dominant but can easily switch to a sub in order to teach someone else.

Tip #45: You can enlist the help of another Dom or sub.

This is not as kinky as it sounds. Believe it or not, there is such a thing as "tagging along" and conversing with an experienced Dom or sub without actually cheating or having kinky fun with them. Most of them are happy to share their knowledge and give tips on how to improve one's craft.

A Dom may allow another Dom to come with him while he trains a sub, or a sub can simply watch a scene unfolding. You can even interview them "out of character" and find out what they personally do to keep things interesting and erotic.

Tip #46: You can "outsource" your Dom / sub needs.

This is the most drastic action and is not for all tastes, but it does work for a small part of the population. One partner stays married but has a Dom outside of the marriage bedroom.

It's an unusual dynamic but for swingers and cuckolding types it addresses a problem in a simple way. They get to keep the intimacy of marriage, while still seeking the eroticism they lack in life because their partner cannot satisfy their craving.

This type of contact must be negotiated and one shouldn't pressure the other one. In most cases, people who seek extreme answers—and who are jealous and insecure by nature—are doomed to end their relationship with this radical behavior.

The couples who actually do make it work have found ways to cope with jealousy or lessen it, and are not motivated by revenge or by the desire to cheat. They simply trust each other to a high degree and have figured out a way to mutually benefit from another lover.

Some unsatisfied lovers will actually suggest swinging or Dom/sub relationships specifically to destroy the relationship or marriage. They know what they're doing and know that their partner can't handle it, but that's the ignition they need to do something they've wanted to do for a long time.

So you can certainly understand why volunteering help from outside the marriage can be a great risk, and shouldn't be taken lightly.

Both partners must be united in trust and in their list of wants—namely that it's just for sex or BDSM purposes, and that emotional affairs are out of the question.

Then again, among some in the lifestyle, emotional and physical affairs are completely fine. Let's take a glimpse into the non-traditional in our next chapter.

Chapter 9: What to Do if You Can't Find any Doms or Subs to Play With

As you probably know by now, there are many unusual relationships in the BDSM lifestyle that break tradition. Some of them are:

- Threesomes (Inviting another person into one's bed, but not necessarily with a BDSM goal in mind)

- Swinging (a couple having sex with another couple, usually in the same room or in the same house)

- Cuckolding or sharing (a couple inviting a third person, usually a Sub or Dom, into their bed; one usually watches)

- Open marriage (the freedom to sleep with other people at any point, but still stayed)

- Orgies (Indiscriminate sex, with multiple partners and anything goes)

- BDSM parties (similar to orgies except that instead of sex, light spanking or light foreplay may be all that's allowed)

Within these nontraditional relationships are room for many variances beyond just short-term affairs or strictly sexual unions. For example, there are exhibitionists who only like to put on a show, such as in an adult theater, rather than actively seek out sex partners. Some couples may only want online role play sex or phone sex.

Then there are those couples interested in something more emotional and meaningful than just a series of one nightstands. In addition to wanting a regular and ongoing sex partner, they may even want a live-in boyfriend or girlfriend. These are known as polyamorous households. These relationships may involve multiple subs under one Dom or they may be all equals.

All of these relationships have a few things in common: they put great emphasis on communication, loyalty (and confessing every secret), mutual respect and honesty.

These relationships are also characterized by having respect for each other and the roles assigned. The reason these couples have found room to play with other people is because they are having all of their needs met without complaint.

They have found a way to meet each individual's needs within the living situation, even if it consists of three or more people.

This is a major point of all relationships; fulfilling expectations created. Even monogamous and vanilla relationships have "contracts," though they are only implied. Once a partner starts breaking that contract of agreements, they violate the existing trust.

Tip #47: Visit a swinger club or BDSM club with your partner to feel out whether this is for you or not.

If you are unsure about expanding your sexual options within a committed relationship, you can always go visit a club with the sole intention of conversing. You don't have to participate or even watch. Some couples simply go, sit down and make small talk. Other couples may approach them and just say hello.

Then they decide whether they are intrigued by the idea of pursuing more, or if the experience was simply too nerve-wracking to continue.

Some couples may avoid crowds and simply flirt with strangers in bars to see where the attraction goes. However, it is important to note...

Tip #48: Meeting random people for sexual adventures can be dangerous.

Just as you once had a filter for screening people when you were single, you should be even more cautious if you are looking for play as a couple. Dealing with potential psychopaths, creeps, deviants and sex offenders and other "crazies" is precisely why it may SEEM as if many in the casual sex community avoid playing with people they don't know.

A well-known BDSM website called FetLife recently closed their doors to new members, indicating that the best way to get involved in BDSM is to meet someone who's already into it. Doesn't seem fair to newcomers, but from the perspective of those in the community, it's a precaution they feel they have to take.

This may cause you stress, whether as a couple or single person, as it may seem that there are far too many single men looking to be Doms than there are subs looking for a relationship.

There are two options to consider.

Tip #49: Attend a "Munch," which is a BDSM-social function that involves simply meeting people in normal situations, outside the element of sexuality or kink.

There are meetups groups of this type in almost every major city. In addition to local meet up groups there are also forums and dating sites that can provide you with a "match." This will be more efficient than surfing Facebook or Craigslist, where the psychos and drama queens are many and the serious BDSM players are hard to find.

Tip #50: Be very careful about trusting people you just met, in regards to sexual hygiene.

So let's say you found someone sane and attractive and want to explore your options with them as a couple. It may be old-fashioned to say this, but it's more true now than ever before. *Don't have sex without a condom.* This includes oral sex and other forms of foreplay. Ideally, the threesome or swinging foursome should be tested to remove all doubt. But if that's not doable wearing a condom is shrewd thinking.

If you're going to engage in cunnilingus then a dental dam or even plastic wrap has been suggested by such sources as the Centers for Disease Control and Prevention and AIDS.gov. However, make sure the wrap is not microwavable, as these do have small pores that could compromise safety.

One recent estimate suggests that one in four people in New York City may have herpes. It's always best to err on the side of caution and not take risks with new people you meet. Even if you get to know some body, you can't be sure of their sexual history — especially since many lovers today are unaware that they have STDs like HPV or gonorrhea.

Tip #51: If you can't seem to find anyone to join you in your kinky play, then it's time to start teaching others what you know.

The neat thing about role playing, kink and BDSM is that even if you can't find the Dom or the sub of your dreams, you can always have fun teaching a new lover what you do know. Since BDSM lifestyle is so variable from person to person, you can rest assured that everyone has some sort of kink they would respond to if you (or you and your partner) show them the way.

They might not even know they have this kink yet, which is why they need a good teacher to show them how their body and mind works. Although you do have to take things very slow with a novice, you may be surprised at what you discover in terms of suppressed desires.

Speaking of kinky desires, it's time to discuss the elephant in the room. Or shall we say, "the whole chicken." What do you do if your partner's sexual kink is WAY over the line of good taste? Let's tread lightly to the next chapter.

Chapter 10: What If Your Partner's Kink is Too Weird or Dangerous?

Now this scenario happens fairly often. You're both going at it and things are nice and steamy. All of a sudden your partner bursts out with an idea that's totally out in left field. Not only is it weird and mood-killing but it may even bother you morally.

Yes, it's true, when you give someone permission to unleash their wildest thoughts you do sometimes get some shocking revelations.

It may be very disturbing if the thoughts you hear involve what most people consider unnatural sex or some sort of deviant lifestyle. With the exception of a few taboos, which we'll discuss later in this chapter, you usually have nothing to worry about.

Some of the most disturbing fantasies are actually quite normal in terms of the huge population that has them. Rape fantasies are among the top fantasies of all women, and many men, as is blackmail, coercion, and humiliation—perhaps even slapping a woman, calling her filthy names and treating her like an object.

These fantasies are very common and usually indicate control issues, which again are normal and within the "radius" of acceptable mainstream behavior.

Now sometimes a partner may take a fantasy and turn it too far right or left, such as with self-cutting, burning or electric shock, beating or bruising, and perhaps even more traumatic mutilation of the body. Some women have fantasies of being impregnated by someone other than their partner. Some men fantasize about beating a slave girl and injuring her. Some people like water sports or scat play, which may be repulsive to a vanilla lover or even a BDSM enthusiast.

Yes, your initial reaction may be shock or even disgust, but don't start divorce proceedings just yet. After all, you were the one that asked your partner to be honest. If you make him or her feel shame, right after they trusted you with their most guarded secret, communication will suffer greatly.

It's okay to be surprised and admit surprise. But don't judge them and don't react in anger or outrage. You can admit that you don't understand a person's fetish. If this is the case, then don't kill the conversation out of fear.

Tip #52: Accept their fantasy, commend their honesty and then ask them to explain it.

One of the most fascinating aspects of fetishes is why they happen to otherwise well-adjusted and happy people. In the majority of cases, even the strangest kinks all come from somewhere. Usually these attractions to the taboo and danger come from childhood trauma.

An easy example is spanking. If a child was spanked and grew up terrified of spankings from his/her parents, then he/she is more likely to find spanking erotic. And the more realistic, and bizarre scenarios, the better. It's not because the person is a weirdo or a pervert. It's simply the human mind and body reacting to something that happened in the past and manifesting those ambivalent feelings in sexual expression.

How about men who like to wear panties and bras? They may have found that wearing women's clothing gives them a feeling of security and inhibition. They feel safer wearing them because of a strong connection to their mother; these feelings stemming from childhood are usually very innocent.

Tip #53: As with all negotiation, your partner volunteers the fetish and the fantasy and then you make a compromise.

Understand that when most people offer a fantasy they know it can never happen in real life. It's the partner's task to find something close or similar to what the other is thinking. They have to find a compromise as a couple.

In the case of an orgy, for example, if the wife is not comfortable doing that, she can decide what level of experimentation she wants to pursue. Level 2 would be sharing a vivid fantasy about a threesome. Level 3 might be to watch porn or read erotica about the experience. Level 4 would be to flirt with a new person and experiment with the feelings. Level 10 would be an orgy just like the man described, but she might never want to go that far.

The same is true in dealing with most fetishes and strange attractions that your partner may bring up. Let's say your partner has an unusually harsh rape fantasy. She wants to be tied up, slapped, choked and impregnated by a stranger. That's never going to happen in real life, you decide. But what can you do to give her some of her fantasy, to the extent that you're comfortable with it and she's enjoying it?

You could dress up like stranger and tie her to a bed. You can lightly choke her or slap her. Or you could write a story or video tape your role play so she can watch it later. There are all sorts of ways to give her a similar experience without endangering her by pursuing something that in real life may be too much to handle.

Tip #54: In cases of extreme fetishism, resist the urge to panic and condemn your partner.

Find out where the fetish comes from and if it's possible that it comes from a peaceful place, not a violent one. Find common ground, where possible.

Naturally, some partners are very squeamish when discussing extreme sexual fantasies, such as those involving bestiality, pedophilia or murderous gore fantasies. It's easy to understand why discussing these things would be troubling.

But again, your first reaction should be to listen and ask your partner to explain on why the attraction is there. Your goal now is to find common ground. You're not relating to your partner's extreme fantasy as is—you're negotiating. You're finding things within that fantasy that you can agree upon and work with.

For instance, bestiality is a bad thing in real life. But there is a whole subculture of "furries" that is pretty big at comic book conventions. People dress up as characters that are anthropomorphic and enjoy visualizing the alien-human sex going on. Or they may like the werewolf or werebear fantasy, which is not true bestiality—it's something in between normal and weird.

In other words, it's something fairly easy to work with and not get all worked up about. There is nothing wrong with the partner that dabbles into the taboo, it's not nearly the same thing as a person actually attracted to animals.

The same thing is true of age play. At first, the confession of having underage sex may be shocking to hear from your partner. But if you resist being easily offended and instead get to the root of the attraction, you may find an interesting discussion.

Sometimes people might have underage fantasies because:

- They had a crush on a teacher as a child

- They have a spanking and mommy/daddy fetish

- They want to be pampered and disciplined like a baby

- They like playing innocent, childlike and easily corruptible—in their adult body

- They enjoy feeling guilty for sexual behavior; it's a pleasurable pain

- They fondly remember their childhood where boys or girls were much easier to talk to than today

These are all perfectly rational reasons why someone might confess an underage fantasy, and it really has nothing to do with child abuse. You can role play as consenting adults and use underage scenarios in the privacy of your own home. Some men really enjoy breastfeeding fantasies and some women enjoy pretending to be a high school student forced into sex by their teacher.

You can't get in trouble for this, so as long as you don't truly have violent tendencies towards children.

Tip #55: If it is blatant and obvious that your partner may have violent pedophiliac desires, professional counseling is the best option.

Give your partner the benefit of the doubt unless you actually get a confession. Don't read into something that may not be there. If your partner admits the attraction to younger lovers, cheerleader outfits, schoolgirl or boy role play, that's nothing to be concerned about. However, if he / she admits strong sexual feelings towards a child and admits the desire to rape, that is obviously grounds for getting professional help.

However, that is a VERY rare scenario and it will be only a very small minority of the population that has to deal with that. Even in that worst case scenario, remember that counseling can help and there are many people that have this condition, who never act upon their feelings. Professional counseling can help patients to control their impulses.

Tip #56: When it comes to murder fantasies, don't take things so bloody seriously.

It's understandable why murder fantasies are shocking and scary at first. But understand this is probably more common than you think. Why just consider the mainstream popularity of movies like Saw, Hostel and Paranormal Activity. Believe it or not, old Hitchcock movies were once considered extreme. We've certainly come a long way in our world of make-believe.

It's safe to say most fantasies involving horror or sadism are probably not going to be cause for alarm. Rape is a common fantasy and yes, some taboo fantasies may involve murdering a person—in essence, assuming the role of Freddy Krueger, Jason or Michael Myers.

This is not necessarily cause for alarm. Many people flirt with the idea of danger and it doesn't mean they are real life psychopaths. They probably enjoy toying with dangerous fantasies for the same reason we all like to watch horror movies—the adrenaline rush and the erotic fear it plays upon.

Now that said, if you feel uncomfortable with murder in your sexual fantasies, you do have the right to say NO, and to offer a compromise that's less severe. Instead of murder, you can substitute something like, pretending to knock out the victim or pretending to beat them until they faint. Some couples might not be offended at the idea of one "murdering" the other and pretending to play dead. It's another "rape" fantasy that sounds more disturbing than it actually is in role play.

It's really up to you as an individual to see how far you want to take the weirdness and fetishism. Rest assured, you are not alone in this particular kink, but obviously, for safety reasons it is not really something people talk about in the open because it is a fantasy that is not for all tastes and can very easily offend other people.

What If Your Own Fantasies Scare You?

What if you're the one with the freaky fantasies and are concerned about scaring your partner to death? It's easy to understand your dilemma; if you want the taboo desperately but fear confessing the truth, it can be stressful. It may be even worse if she knows the fantasy you have but really doesn't respond to it. That may make you feel perverted. What can you do?

Tip #57: Don't fight, don't suppress. Confess openly and explain your feelings on the matter.

Explaining your attractions and obsessions to your partner may actually help a lot. When doing so, don't brag. Talk about the feelings you have. Admit the shame if you have it, and express your desire to talk and be honest. Chances are she will listen and offer her compromise, which may excite you in brand new ways.

Recognize that most sexual obsessions involve negative emotions like anxiety, guilt and shame. The person rationalizes he/she must be evil for having them, when in actuality, it's mostly symptoms of Obsessive-compulsive Disorder (OCD).

Having unnatural or even unspeakable thoughts is not any indication that you're warped or disturbed. They usually are, like dreams, related to something going on in your subconscious.

A lot of men have strange sexual thoughts about their mothers. It certainly doesn't mean the man has a literal Oedipus complex. It probably means though, that there are issues stemming from childhood that he finds attractive. He may have a mom fetish, for other moms or may want to pretend to be a child, being sexually assaulted by her. It's really about his ego and id, and not about any sort of deviancy.

The real problem is that rather than confess these unusual feelings and get it out in the open, many people suppress them entirely. That only makes the thought more intense, more troubling and bringing more stress to the person thinking it. People with OCD may even isolate themselves because of the guilt.

For example, some obsessive sexual thoughts you may have could involve:

- Cheating on your spouse

- Losing control and trying to rape someone

- Wanting to expose yourself

- Wanting sex with a same sex partner

- Having unprotected sex or other dangerous fantasies

- Sex with corpses or blood and cutting play

- Sex with religious persons; priests, nuns, or even with god deities themselves

- Sex with family members

- Violent or murderous fantasies

What might be of comfort to you is to know that…

Tip #58: Understand that usually people are AFRAID of the deviant fetish; they are not compelled by it.

It's the difference between fearing something (and maybe using its overtones to enjoy better sex) and actually wanting to do something dangerous or unhealthy, which would be a compulsion.

Consider an example. One question that doctors ask pedophiles is "If you could get away with a crime would you do it?" The pedophiles always say yes. The people tormented by OCD always answer No, of course not. That's the difference.

While counseling can help people suffering from OCD, usually when it comes to having "disturbing sexual thoughts" there is nothing to be concerned about. It's only if the OCD affects your life to the point where you are a threat to yourself or others. If you can't function normally then it's a problem.

Tip #59: If it's a fetish that's not hurting anybody, then by all means tell your partner and see what he/she can do to help you break new taboos.

Having an understanding partner is almost better than therapy in cases where there is only light fetishism. If you have the hots for young and virile bodies, then there's nothing wrong with your wife dressing up in a cheerleader outfit. There's nothing wrong with a woman pretending to seduce a female student. There's nothing wrong with a man pretending to break in the house and tie his wife up and then blindfold her.

In many BDSM heavy households, you may see even more extreme scenarios. Like a younger couple having sex with young twenty-year olds, or a well-endowed man pleasuring a man's wife.

What about the wife that knows her husband has bisexual fantasies and so she indulges him with gay porn? What about the wife that goes one step further and allows her husband to have sex with another man while she watches?

These scenarios might be considered aberrant by some, but they are fairly normal within context. If exploring these taboos can help alleviate obsessive sexual thoughts, then it's far better to explore them rather than keep suppressing them and feeling guilt.

Tip #60: If you or your partner has "soft limits" to explore, then use concepts of "cognitive behavioral therapy" to help him or her come out of that shell.

This means that rather than spring something scary upon your partner, you slow things down by gradually introducing new stimuli that only hints at their taboo fear. If there's a taboo that makes them afraid but excited, then practice getting gradually closer and closer.

Take small steps until he/she learns not to be afraid of the thought but attentive. Now he or she becomes gradually used to the new sensation, thinking about these once terrifying thoughts. The partner learns to deal with the feelings and realize that the thoughts are harmless, if still eccentric. But now he/she is in a place to explore this attraction safely and think about why it's appealing.

Tip #61: The key is to STOP fighting and resist the urge to say NO.

This is suppressed behavior and the OCD thoughts will only intensify if you refuse to entertain the notion.

This is why exploring these taboos is ultimately freeing and even healthy—compared to suppressing your instincts.

If you need help, then you'll get help if and when you reach that point. But don't assume you're a terrible person just because you have obsessive sexual thoughts. Sexuality is inherently connected to who a person really is and what their desires are in life. You don't always understand where strange erotic thoughts come from, but the discovery will always be enlightening…and in some cases, very sexy if your partner can help you exploit it.

In our next chapter, we're going to discuss a less controversial but just as interesting a topic: the concept of erotic peaking—specifically, the idea that a person can orgasm just because they are instructed to do so by a Dom. Is this really possible?

Chapter 11: What about Orgasming on Command?

Is it really possible to orgasm on command or is this just a crazy bondage fantasy?

It's true, but it may require a lot more effort than just willpower alone. Subs must be trained to be orgasmic on command. Once they give power to the Dom, they have already given their body permission to orgasm. It's a bit of a mental anchor that the Dom and sub create in intensive training. Since orgasms are mostly mental, it's understandable how they can be "summoned" through anchoring words and actions.

Subs who can orgasm on command can easily orgasm during sex and in masturbation, so it's not as if this is a "Cure" for a woman who has trust issues or sexual fears. This is a more "advanced" game that some subs play because they are so easily orgasmic.

Tip #62: The Dom's goal is to replace the fear of not orgasming with the fear of orgasming without permission.

This is actually an attitude that the Dom can instill in the sub with practice.

The Dom usually instructs the sub to not orgasm without his permission. He can say yes or no, and get her craving them. This gives the Dom the privilege of making the sub "edge" over and over without orgasming—because he hasn't given the word. He keeps the sub just on the brink of orgasm and tortures her, until he's ready to give her permission. This makes the sub's orgasm—which by now is much desired and imminent—much easier to trigger.

Tip #63: The power of suggestion, hypnotic reaction in the sub, can help to induce an orgasm on command.

After much practice, giving suggestions and "observations" about the sub (but not actual commands) and how close she is to orgasm can also help prepare her body for the response. By the time he actually tells her to orgasm, she has been eagerly awaiting the climax.

Many Doms and subs claim that a sub must give ownership of her body and orgasm to the Dom, for the psychological conditioning to work. This is not only a ritual but also a means to prevent the sub from masturbating or orgasming without the Dom present.

Tip #64: During training, when the Dom brings the sub to orgasm, you should create a trigger word.

This anchoring technique associates erotic feelings with a single word, (preferably a word that has no meaning outside in the real world) that acts as the one trigger that gives full permission for her to come.

The Dom actually trains the sub in advance to connect feelings of orgasm with a word and or touch, which connects stimuli to a single moment. The body can be trained to auto-respond to the "anchoring" word or gesture.

Oftentimes Doms will tell subs to mastur-bate on their own just so subs can learn how to quickly and easily make themselves come. Then the next step is edging and reaching a point of near orgasm that will continually stay in the sub's mind but not crossing that thresh-old without permission.

Tip #65: Edging is key because it trains the sub to focus on not having an orgasm rather than having one.

Respectively reaching a state of near orgasm but not giving yourself permission to come will create more tension and bring her closer to near orgasm without actually experiencing it.

This challenges the mind and the body and reconditions the sub's ideas of who's in control, even if it's on a subconscious level. Some Doms even get multiple orgasms based on the idea of suggestion and the suppression of orgasm.

The training time will vary of course and the Dom should always make it a point to be reassuring to her, to reach her subconscious and not pressure her about what he wants. He's giving her permission to orgasm. He may even talk to her, using mere words to try and trigger a sexual response based only on the sub's accumulated lust and the desire to obey a person she trusts. The more gratitude and care a Dom shows, in conditioning and in aftermath, the more response he can expect when he gives the order.

All this talk of orgasming on command and repetitive peaking may make you wonder if you're really unleashing a great evil upon this world! That's an interesting subject actually, as we consider supposedly the dark side of erotic taboo—the state of "frenzy" where your partner or you become insatiably horny and obsessed with breaking more taboos. Is this a real issue in BDSM or is it exaggerated?

Chapter 12: What is "Frenzy" and Can You Become Desensitized?

The idea of "Frenzy", or Sub-Frenzy, is basically an out of control sub that has been stimulated beyond what she can handle. It's also described as a consuming desire to experience every kind of kink imaginable and do so as often as possible. Isn't this just enthusiasm or horny behavior? Is it really a dangerous condition?

The only real danger is when an out of control sub is paired with a Dom that can't control her. The Dom's job is to protect the sub and make sure she can deal with her desires and enflamed impulses in a safe way.

If a Dom notices that a sub is getting too addicted to the sessions, his response should never be to abandon her, but to guide her back to a manageable state of mind.

In BDSM lifestyle, it is observed that subs who are in a sub-frenzy state tend to make big mistakes because of their enthusiasm, like playing too intensely with someone they just met, playing too often and not giving it enough healing time, agreeing to anything and to everyone, no demands or questions, just acceptance (even out of character).

These situations can be harmful because without a strong Dom the sub could put herself in a dangerous situation with unsavory characters.

Tip #66: Remember that the sub may not be capable of making rational decisions at various points of the session. When adrenaline and endorphin rush is involved, it can affect emotion and logic.

Endorphin release happens after the body is placed under unusual stress and adrenaline is the fight or flight response that's even more intense. These altered states can happen after prolonged spanking or other pain-pleasure activities.

Stuck in euphoria, (not to mention the "drop" that occurs after) can be a very vulnerable state and the sub must be coddled and supported during this highly emotional state. Failure to tend to their needs could result in unpredictable emotional outbursts. Which brings us to the subject of…*When Subs Go Bad*.

Tip #67: If you're a Dom, avoid subs that drop all sorts of red flags. Gather knowledge and be alert.

While this book is centered on couples, this lesson bears repeating even in this context. Why? Because even if your partner is a loving and trustworthy BDSM player, they are still subject to the extreme emotions and sensations of endorphinal rush.

Whether it's your wife, girlfriend or a random stranger you met, be aware of the warning signs so that you can put the brakes on BEFORE you start taking her into deep sub space and high emotion.

Subs that are moving too fast may show rather obvious signs of addiction, out of control mood swings, or taking dangerous risks all in the name of sexual exploration. As a Dom partner, even if it's your wife or girlfriend, you must be strong and smart and realize if she's moving too fast. (He or she of course, but the Dom is typically used in the male persona)

Tip #68: Beware of an unhappy sub, whom you've failed to direct.

She can turn against you pretty quickly, blaming you for every unhappy thought or sensation that happens. This is much worse in singles BDSM dating, but it's not unthinkable that it would happen in a relationship.

Misunderstandings cause major problems and can really upset a sub if she feels vulnerable and the Dom doesn't protect her, or make her feel secure, the way she's counting on. Worst case scenario, usually in the singles scene, she accuses him of being a dangerous Dom / rapist.

More likely scenario in a committed relationship, she just resents you for not being there when she needed a strong arm to support her and she closes her mind off to future experimentation. So yes, it happens and it emphasizes the point to:

Tip #69: Always be emotionally available, before, during and after the scene.

Nothing is more important than making sure your sub or life partner is cared for, not even the intensity of the scene. If you sense she is vulnerable or in need of reassurance then ask her a question. Check in on her and make sure she's ready to keep going.

Tip #70: Learning your partner helps you to avoid scenarios that might excite her too much or leave her in subdrop.

Subdrop refers to the crash that happens after a state of euphoria. This can be a depressive state and if that happens, don't expect any more kinky fun for a while. To avoid leaving your sub unattended (mentally and emotionally, not just physically) ask questions and discuss the scene after it ends.

Don't take for granted that you're together outside of the BDSM fantasy. If you're introducing your partner to new emotions then you have to be there for her after the session to keep her warm, make sure she feels loved, and instill the "training" in her, which teaches her to keep trusting you.

Some Doms find it useful to keep a journal of what transpires or to ask the sub to keep a journal for reference. Counting on your own memory may be problematic.

This leads us to the question of the day, or really the question of the YEAR, and what's bound to be one everyone's mind who ever doubted the safety of BDSM.

Can you get desensitized?

In other words, this simply means an extended state of sub frenzy where you crave more taboo breaking, more and more until you become a sex crazed animal!

Is there any truth to this?

This rumor stems from mostly religious objection to sexual exploration, and it's founded in fear of the unknown. Understand that most objections to sexual adventure comes, not from a fear of losing all inhibitions and becoming "frenzied," but of discovering something new about yourself. Something that may be in conflict with a strict religious upbringing.

Therefore, the easy answer is does BDSM desensitize you? Yes, to the same old sexual experiences you've already had and have grown tired of. But there is no evidence suggesting that you're taking a "gateway drug" to new levels of perversity.

Escalation is mostly a myth because logic tells us that what we crave, we seek more of; when we have had enough, we avoid it. So if you find that experimenting with some kinky activity turns you on, by all means pursue it.

Progress onward at your own pace. At some point, with the guidance of your partner, you may discover that you have gone too far. You surpassed a boundary and it made you feel afraid or sickened for some reason.

Now you've reached your personal threshold. You can turn what was a soft limit into a hard limit. Or you can decide to try to conquer the new threshold again, by taking things much slower.

But the thing of it is, you get to decide how much is too much. Why should you deprive yourself of going a little farther just because you're afraid that you might find out something new about yourself—your kinks and even some latent desires? Kinks and bucket list wishes you never even knew existed inside of you?

Sometimes people even discover that doing something more than once may produce different emotional reactions; sometimes good, sometimes not so good. But it's worth trying again.

The truth is, variance is the best way to ensure maximum arousal. When someone watches porn, for example, he may become desensitized to R rated sex scenes on TV because they don't give him the images he craves. But when he finds the threshold of XXX, he doesn't want "more." He is not drawn to violence or rape. He simply tires of the sexual images for a while and then comes back for more stimulation when he's ready. In that manner…

Tip #71: Understand that sexual exploration is not a runaway car, certain to take you off a cliff.

It's a "car" that you drive, and one that you have control over, as well as your partner.

Another point to keep in mind is that curiosity is what powers eroticism. It's not perversity, it's not demonism or any negative emotion. It's simply curiosity; we explore it and select what taboos are interesting.

Tip #72: You will find that as you grow, your interests will change. Accept it and be flexible.

Like your eating habits, your sexual interests will change over time. It's not because of desensitization. It's because you as a person change gradually throughout your life. Sometimes you change in subtle ways, sometimes in more peripheral ways.

After experiencing something sexually powerful and memorable, you may even find that you are either more inclined to push yourself into experimental territory, or less inclined to go in certain directions.

Some people experiment with flirting with third parties and then retreat back to a safe spot because they don't like the jealousy issues that arise. That's their limit. They reach it, and they have no regrets.

Experiences only become traumatic if you let it ride that far out. That's why taking it slow is always essential. Not just for comfort reasons and trust, but also so that you don't risk trauma from trying something completely out of your element too soon—and suffering negative emotions from it.

But in general, your tastes and desires will change with age so be open to it. Don't consider chasing taboos and finding new ways to pique your curiosity and that of your lover's obscene. You cannot become desensitized to something pleasurable.

Nobody wants to have sex in the exact same manner every day. They want variety and that's really all that BDSM play is about. Finding varieties that we enjoy—not seeking out extremes that terrify us.

Speaking of aging, what happens when we attempt to confine the kinky and fantastical with real life? Specifically, family, children and in-laws? Oh boy, get ready for Chapter 13.

Chapter 13: How to Balance Being a Kinkster and a Parent

A kinkster has to grow up at some point and think of their children, right?

Well, not necessarily. This seems to be a cliché among many parents, particularly in strict religious communities, who equate "kinky fun" or BDSM with wild behavior.

Of course, within any kind of sexual exploration there is the potential for dangerous behavior. And it's true that as parents you do not want to expose your children to a hectic and morally ambiguous environment.

But is kinkster fun really all that bad?

What are we actually afraid of anyway, that our children will discover our chains and leather whips? Or that mom, dad and Uncle James will be a bad influence on children?

This is an issue that's really simple to solve if you think about it.

Tip #73: Use traditional wording and concepts in casual talk, rather than try to use words that are too complex or confusing to a young mind.

No, you don't explain your BDSM fantasies or lifestyle choices to your children. But you're not ashamed of them either. Obviously, vanilla parents would not go into great detail when explaining the joys of sex to their children. In fact, most parents usually just deliver a very concise, very scientific explanation of what sex involves, when their children have curiosity about it.

In terms of vocabulary, it's easy to see why you should use familiar wording and not try to overwhelm their minds with new age thoughts. Mom and dad don't have a "date" with someone else tonight. They are simply meeting with friends. Dad doesn't have a mom-baby fetish; he just has private time with mom. Mom doesn't like to be "tied up" she's just "playing with dad."

It's never really a pleasant conversation when parents decide to have the talk about sex with their children, because of some of the questions being asked.

However, the idea that you should be ashamed of your kinky preferences and dispose of them completely before having children is a bit ridiculous. That's like saying, you shouldn't have sex once you give birth because of the possibility of your children walking in on you. That's absurd and children are not going to be traumatized even if they accidentally see something happening.

Just as when a child walks in on his parents in bed, you simply stop what you're doing and tend to his needs. In the worst case scenario, you would ask him to leave while you take care of your predicament (such as, if you're tied up or something like that).

Yes, if the child seemed bothered or confused, you would take the time to say you were just playing. In most cases, children will forget what they see and go about their day.

Otherwise, all you really have to do is be discreet about your vocabulary.

There's no logical reason why your sex life should be non-existent just because you're raising children. Whether you want to put strict limits on "visitors" coming over or doing anything in plain sight, obviously is another issue altogether. Children may not be able to comprehend open marriages or pain infliction so avoid any imagery that might be too much unless you lock the door behind you.

Tip #74: Teaching children boundaries as relates to asking questions about private matters is just a life lesson they need to learn. Explain to them that your sex life is your private business.

You do want to prevent showing them too much—such as multiple lovers or other unusual fetishistic practices. Avoid combining the kinkiest aspects of your life with family routines while children are around and watching.

If they ask more detailed sexual questions, then you do have the right to say that it's private and not appropriate conversation until the child grows older.

Tip #75: Many couples into the swinging lifestyle or BDSM do have children but they make it a point to play somewhere else besides the home. Someone else hosts so that they run no risk of waking or alarming children.

It's a good precedent to keep your family life separate from your kinky life as much as possible, especially when exploring brand new taboos. This may also mean hiding the truth from family members (parents, aunts, uncles) that might not understand.

If conservative-minded people hear about your kinky lives, they might worry about the welfare of your children. Simple solution: never tell them, unless they admit their kinky lives to you first. Otherwise, it's none of their business, just as it's not the business of your children. Your private sex life is between you and your partner, and no one else.

The question is, is it moral to be having polyamorous affairs or exploratory fun with other people besides your partner if you have children?

Obviously, traditionalists feel strongly about a marriage consisting of one man and one woman; claiming that it helps to stabilize the home environment. This is mostly speculation, because every day there are more gay and lesbian couples adopting children and starting their own families, all of whom turn out fine.

The traditional family model is not always required to raise a stable youth with a good head on his shoulders; just look at how many single mothers raise their children without any serious drawbacks.

The idea that a husband and wife can't be kinky if they are to be "good parents" is outdated. What does matter is the proper management of time.

Tip #76: Good parents do not neglect their children's growing needs; their health, education and moral upbringing.

So as long as you can teach your children what they need to know about how to live, how to make a career, and how to be kind towards others, kinky is really of secondary importance.

Being a good parent DOES involve putting you children's needs ahead of your sexual recreation, obviously. In these instances, naturally, your children's interest would come first:

- No sexy fun until children have a babysitter or are at someone's house who is a trusted friend or family member

- Their material needs are taken care of before your recreational spending

- Their need to talk to a parent is more important than sexual adventures

- Neglecting a child's needs is never excusable, even when in lust or D/s play

And in other instances like these, you would make rational decisions, perhaps even putting your sexual pleasures second on the list, after taking care of family needs. This is responsibility, but this does not mean your sex life is over. Responsibility doesn't mean the end of spontaneous and playful shenanigans.

Besides, you're not going to pass on your kinks to your children because of your ENVI-RONMENT—unless of course you practice free sex in open view, which most couples don't. More than likely any kinks will be passed on through genetics and nothing more. If you're discreet, your children are going to be fine.

The only remaining issue is whether or not you can reconcile the issue on your own. How you can be a kinky parent but a loving and traditional parent in all other areas? Of course, it can be done, and as with all alternative life-styles, the only question to ask yourself is: am I hurting anybody?

Since the idea of sexual experimentation is pleasure (and even the pain of discipline re-sults in pleasure) for many kinky couples the answer is no. You're not hurting anyone, you're merely raising a family while holding on to the best years of your sex life. It's a positive thing.

In fact many couples are heavily stressed from family obligations and may find that sexual adventures in kink may be just what they need to recharge.

Let's consider other personal aspects of BDSM and whether or not it can affect your everyday life.

Chapter 14: Can BDSM Affect a Couple's Relationship?

Sex is merely an extension of our "normal" lives, and so of course any change in our sex lives, for better or worse, affects our attitudes and our daily routines. A boring vanilla sex life, or a completely sexless life, can affect the way you act and your outlook on life. The same is true of having a kinkier sex life. Yes, it will start to show.

If you both enjoy the taboo exploration then you will be healthier, happier, less tempted to cheat, and generally a more productive person. Many in the lifestyle confess that the kinkier relationships were more satisfying than the vanilla ones, and probably due to the fact that BDSM means excellent communication.

Vanilla sex doesn't require great communication to exist. It's just there. Herein lies the problem. The more "chocolate" a vanilla sex life becomes, the more communication increases, and the more pleasure a searching couple will find.

What can happen is that a person can experiment with BDSM and become very attracted to the new feelings and sensations and NOT desire to go back to vanilla sex. Is this dangerous?

In theory, no, because the taboo attraction is what the person wants. It's not really a physical addiction, but a mental realization that you want more now, now that your mind has been expanded.

Will this change your life? Possibly, and that is why many couples decide to take it slow and eventually STOP at a point before the experimentation takes them into a new lifestyle. A couple may decide they never want a threesome in real life, and so they will stop escalating. On the other hand if a couple decides they enjoy sharing multiple partners, this will cause a change in their lives and they must prepare for that.

Most BDSM experienced players state that the most common problem they see is that one partner wants to be kinky and the other partner doesn't, or wants to stay at a very low level of kink.

Some even quote scientific studies (http://www.livescience.com/34832-bdsm-healthy-psychology.html) stating that kinksters score better on overall mental health than vanilla lovers. This makes sense, given that vanilla lovers tend to suppress desire, whereas kinksters explore it; they reach new levels of contentment, excitement and general happiness for their lifestyle.

Tip #77: Set limits on where you do not want to go, and where you go so that your partner will always respect those limits.

Now if you fear that your partner may escalate and escalate and escalate—eventually surpassing your own threshold for comfort, it may be wise to consider avoiding certain directions and topics early on. Let your partner know your hard and soft limits upfront. There are always ways to get creative and satisfy your mate in a compromise-solution.

There is not an easy answer, however, to steering your mate in the direction of kink and then finding out he/she is more extreme than you are. It may be a stressful situation so proceed with caution, always making it clear from the beginning just how far you want to go and where you do not want to go. Express feelings honestly is the best solution.

How to Turn Real Life Pain into Kinky Redemption

Tip #78: It works best to pursue taboos that make you feel good or that turn negative emotions into something pleasurable.

BDSM is, for all purposes, sexual therapy that you can DIY and benefit from. You literally find areas of your life where there is pain, doubt or confusion and you turn those negative thoughts into something pleasurable. This is when BDSM ceases being about kinky fun and actually becomes mentally healthy for you.

All of us have sources of stress that stem from childhood or traumatic times in our lives. Pursuing fantasies where we "win" and change the bad memory into something erotic is one of the best ways to overcome guilt, self-loathing and memories of exploitation.

Tip #79: Turn negative feelings between you and your partner into something positive and red-hot.

You can actually turn heated moments of argument into kinky fun. There is a process to this of course, and we don't recommend you start spanking your partner right as he/she's yelling at you!

However, keep these tips in mind on how to turn hostile energy into sexual energy:

- Concentrate more on saying why your feelings are provoked

- Don't accuse your partner or use aggressive "pointing" body gestures

- Don't cross your arms; express emotion outward

- Don't shout—just talk with more emotion

- Use "breath" in your words; breathy words and harder breathing

- Don't use personal attacks in the argument

- Take a breather when the negative emotion peaks; fill the pause with energy—now use the adrenaline you've worked up to transform angry energy into sexual energy.

- Let your eyes do the talking; pretend as if this is a first date and then take small SLOW steps forward to your partner. He or she must feel your sexual thoughts, and not think you're moving forward to attack.

- Break your silence, saying something about HOW your partner affects you emotionally. For example, "You're the most stubborn man I've ever met!"

Once your partner realizes your energy has become sexual, you can kiss or take each other's clothes off, having "angry sex" and experiencing yet another taboo feeling.

We've reached the near end of this book, but before we conclude, let's review 10 reasons why BDSM sometimes DOESN'T work—and what these couples are doing wrong.

Chapter 15: 10 Reasons Why BDSM Doesn't Work for Couples—Which You Can Fix

BDSM is bound to "work" and improve your sex life and committed relationship but only if you avoid making emotional, careless and ignorant decisions. We've compiled a list of 10 reasons why couples fail at BDSM, as well as the SOLUTION you need to avoid making those same mistakes.

1. Lack of Communication

The entire basis for good BDSM relations is in honest and raw communication. Hiding your true feelings, all the while wanting power play, could be disastrous. Lack of communicating could also cause problems when the sub wants to go slower, but the Dom partner doesn't get the message. To avoid problems, share everything. It's better to share too much than to hide what you really feel.

2. Dom and/or Sub Partners Not Understanding the Role

A Dom's motivation is not to abuse the sub, nor is the sub's motivation to suffer. A sub has ultimate control over the session and receives pleasure. The Dom's job is to safely guide the sub towards the euphoric state of mind she craves.

3. Moving Too Fast

It's even more important to take things slow when you're already in a committed relationship. As a team of husband and wife or boyfriend and girlfriend you've already built great trust with each other. You can't risk that by trying to go 100 miles per hour in your new sexual adventures. Maintain your partner's trust by taking it slow and putting their comfort over yours.

4. Being Shy About Your Bodies

It's important to conquer body issues, as well as personal trust issues, before pursuing BDSM kink. Otherwise, the sub will not fully trust you and this will hinder the close connection.

5. Not Making Time For It

BDSM play is fairly complex and so it's not practical to think that you can improvise or fit sessions into the weekend, or whenever the mood strikes you. Spontaneous sex may be fun but it doesn't happen nearly as often as you would hope.

6. Improperly Spanking or Tying Up the Sub

Inadvertently hurting the sub by poorly tying their wrists or ankles is a recurring problem among novices, as well as spanking them in ways that hurt and bruise—rather than tingle and sting. Don't over spank a sub in the same section—vary the spot you direct your discipline towards. When spanking him/her, aim for the fleshy cheeks not anywhere else on the backside, which can cause unpleasant pain.

7. Not Going Past the Confession State

Too many couples fast-forward to spanking or fantasies/porn without actually having the honest heart-to-heart talk about what turns them on.

8. Not Being Giving Enough

If one partner is selfishly motivated (as in, I want this fantasy fulfilled at any cost) the intimacy is lost. He is only thinking about his own pleasure and ignoring the desires of his partner. A union between two partners who are both committed to fulfilling each other's fantasy is much stronger.

9. Not Thinking Far Ahead

Not creating hard limits and soft limits can be dangerous. Before you know it, you maybe be dabbling into activities you're not sure how you feel about—or even hitting the state of "Frenzy" where you want anything and everything. Both partners stating at the outset what they want and do NOT want is a good precedent that will define respectful boundaries you both want to keep, for the sake of trust.

10. Giving Up Too Easy When Your Partner Doesn't Want Kink

If your partner doesn't seem enthused at the moment, don't give up on the idea of expanding his/her sexual horizons. Remember that people's desires change and eventually your partner might come around, especially if you keep thinking of new and creative ways to present "kink" into your usual routines.

Conclusion

Here's one last tip to take home:

Bonus Tip: Don't confine sexuality or try to determine all that it must be in your life.

Your sexual persona changes along with you. Rather than trying to limit yourself in terms of "this is all I will ever be" think more along the lines of "this is who I want to be."

While this tip may seem more general than sexual discovery, the point is that by putting limits on how important sex is, you are limiting your pleasure. Now it's one thing to say, "I will never want to have an orgy with strangers!" (A hard limit you set for yourself and your partner) which is understandable.

But if you say, "Sex is just not a big deal to me. It's over in fifteen minutes and it helps me sleep."

In that case, you're putting limits on the benefits of a better sex life. You're dooming yourself to disappointment and intentionally not growing.

The point of sexual discovery is to grow, just as any hobby, or any educational discourse. You don't fully know the benefits of something until you try it—expand the role of study in your life.

Saying that sex is nothing, just bodies clashing and release, misses out on all the spiritual aspects of sex, the emotional intimacy, the powerful emotional surge that can result and the catharsis of making peace with your troubled past. These are just some of the benefits of a more active sex life, not to mention the health benefits and improved levels of happiness.

Sex is a need, at the end of the day, just as are things like entertainment, knowledge, friendship, and family. It may not be as important as food or as a career, but it is definitely one of the great joys in life. By deciding that you have finished exploring sexuality, and are content with the routines, may be depriving yourself of growing as a lover, a person, and ultimately someone driven by passion.

Sex is the "least of it" when you consider how our kinks and erotic taboos are actually fundamental aspects of ourselves—the ego and id of our personalities. The desires we want on an instinctive level, and the desires that we rationalize in day to day life.

Sex, and the exploration of role play, kink and BDSM can help you on your quest to find out who you really are. And that's why it's more important than "just sex".

We hope you have enjoyed reading this book and have a chance to think about some of the tips we reviewed. Maybe you can apply them in your own role plays and activities and have some fun.

Other Books by Elizabeth Cramer

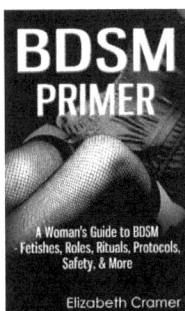

BDSM Primer - A Woman's Guide to BDSM - Fetishes, Roles, Rituals, Protocols, Safety, & More

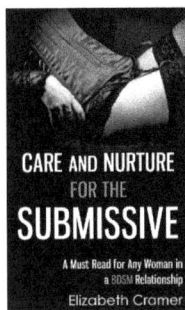

Care and Nurture for the Submissive - A Must Read for Any Woman in a BDSM Relationship

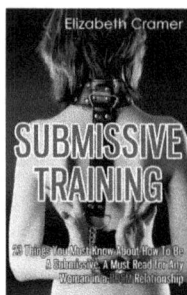

Submissive Training: 23 Things You Must Know About How To Be A Submissive. A Must Read For Any Woman In A BDSM Relationship

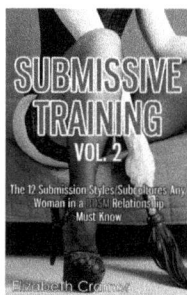

Submissive Training Vol. 2: The 12 Submission Styles/Subcultures Any Woman In A BDSM Relationship Must Know

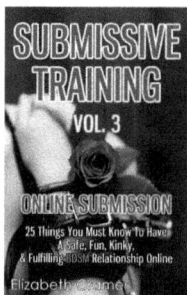

Submissive Training Vol. 3: Online Submission - 25 Things You Must Know To Have A Safe, Fun, Kinky, & Fulfilling BDSM Relationship Online

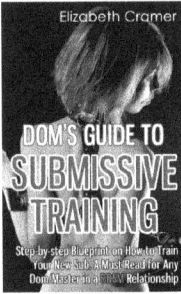

Dom's Guide To Submissive Training: Step-by-step Blueprint On How To Train Your New Sub. A Must Read For Any Dom/Master In A BDSM Relationship

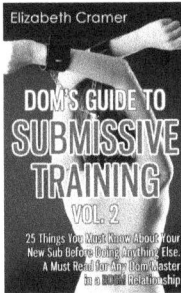

Dom's Guide To Submissive Training Vol. 2: 25 Things You Must Know About Your New Sub Before Doing Anything Else. A Must Read For Any Dom/Master In A BDSM Relationship

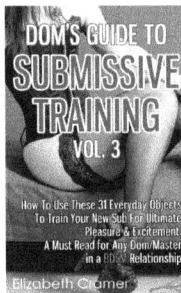

Dom's Guide To Submissive Training Vol. 3: How To Use These 31 Everyday Objects To Train Your New Sub For Ultimate Pleasure & Excitement. A Must Read For Any Dom/Master In A BDSM Relationship

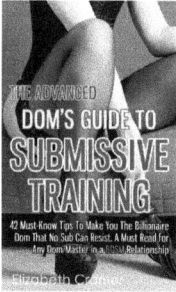

The Advanced Dom's Guide To Submissive Training: 42 Must-Know Tips To Make You The Billionaire DOM That No Sub Can Resist. A Must Read For Any Dom/Master In A BDSM Relationship

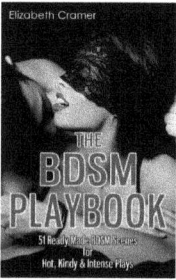

The BDSM Playbook: 51 Ready-Made BDSM Scenes for Hot, Kindy & Intense Plays

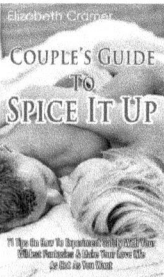

Couple's Guide To Spice It Up: 71 Tips On How To Experiment Safely With Your Wildest Fantasies & Make Your Love Life As Hot As You Want

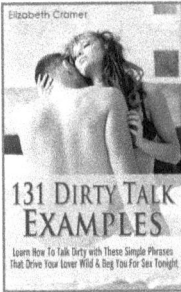

131 Dirty Talk Examples: Learn How To Talk Dirty with These Simple Phrases That Drive Your Lover Wild & Beg You For Sex Tonight

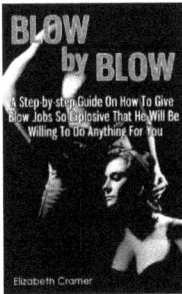

Blow By Blow - A Step-by-step Guide On How To Give Blow Jobs So Explosive That He Will Be Willing To Do Anything For You

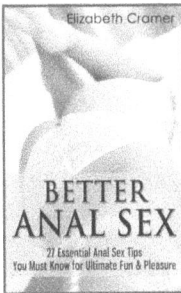

Better Anal Sex - 27 Essential Anal Sex Tips You Must Know for Ultimate Fun & Pleasure

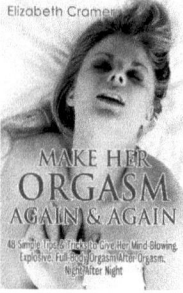

Make Her Orgasm Again and Again: 48 Simple Tips & Tricks to Give Her Mind-Blowing, Explosive, Full-Body Orgasm After Orgasm, Night After Night

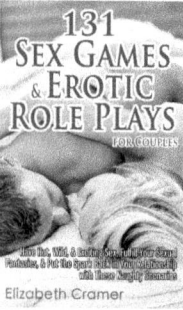

131 Sex Games & Erotic Role Plays for Couples: Have Hot, Wild, & Exciting Sex, Fulfill Your Sexual Fantasies, & Put the Spark Back in Your Relationship with These Naughty Scenarios

9 781724 733061